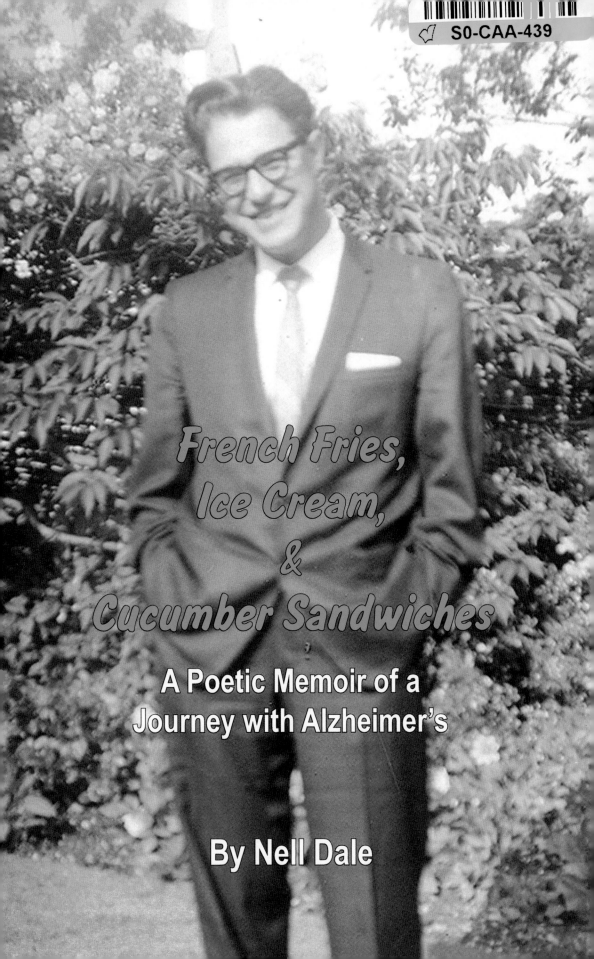

French Fries, Ice Cream, & Cucumber Sandwiches

A Poetic Memoir of a Journey with Alzheimer's

By Nell Dale

To Alfred G. Dale
who allowed me to accompany him on this journey.

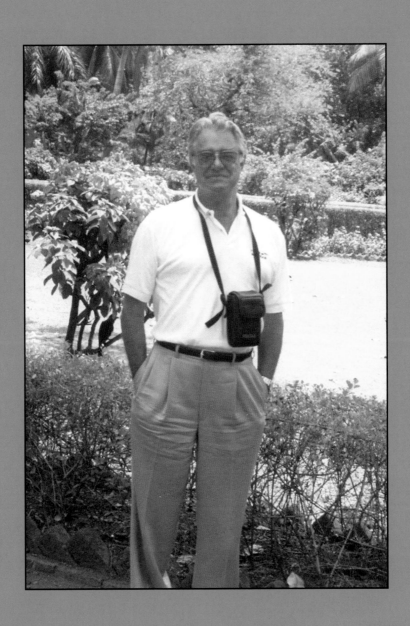

Table of Contents

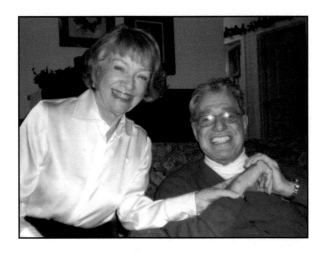

Who Is Left Behind?

After years of a slow, undetected cognitive decline,
five months in and out of the hospital, and a precipitate mental free fall,
Al, our husband and father, was put into Barton House, a loving Alzheimer's facility.
The family has moved on, back to our normal everyday life,
leaving Al behind.

Al now lives in a world in which blue skies are to be marveled at,
and seeing birds on a wire causes him to say "That makes my day."
French fries are viewed with great excitement,
and riding in a car is a wonderful outing.

Is Al really left behind?
He now lives in a world in which only important things matter.
No, Al is not left behind, we are.

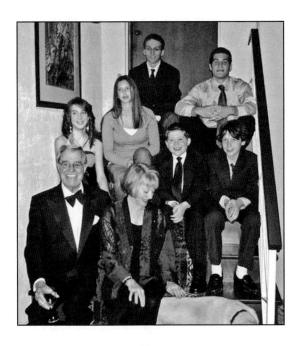

The Appropriate Time

When Al left the rehab hospital, they told me
he would need round-the-clock professional care.
No, I thought;
I can handle this.

I got a nurse for eight hours a day so I could work.
Al didn't want a nurse.
He wanted to watch me work.
He wanted to sit and hold my hand.
He wanted to go for ice cream.
He wanted my complete attention.
I can handle this.
Professional care may be in the future, but not now.

His memory deteriorated rapidly.
He became angry over any change.
He couldn't find the bathroom.
He wouldn't eat.
He was bored, but wouldn't do anything, just
move from room to room restlessly.
Not yet, I thought;
I can handle this.

Then he started wandering.
One night he appeared upstairs, saying
"I have searched the house for the visitors
from overseas and I can't find them anywhere."
There are steps between each room in our house.
Even though I had baby monitors everywhere,
I hadn't heard him wander.
He was no longer safe.

A friend took me to see Barton House,
an Alzheimer's facility where her father had been.
It was small, spotlessly clean, and homey.
The director offered to do a home-visit assessment.
She sat and chatted with us for an hour.
I was stunned at how far he had deteriorated.

Al couldn't remember where he was born,
where he had worked, what he did for a living, or
who the people were in the family photograph.

I put him in Barton House for a week's respite.
We would then reassess the longer term.

The family all met with the staff after a week.
Various members of the staff talked with us,
each saying that Al was adjusting very well.
The activities director said that he particularly
liked playing dominos.
Playing dominos?
No way would my husband play dominos.
Then the light dawned.

I was trying to adjust my world to accommodate him.
I needed to switch my focus from what I could do
to what Al needed.
He needed a safe environment, one created
by people who understood the emotional and cognitive
needs of an Alzheimer's patient.

Although I had gone to the meeting prepared to
bring him home, I knew that now was the appropriate time.

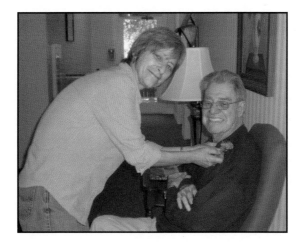

Al's Place

Alzheimer's is a dreadful disease:
It has robbed my husband of his memories,
leaving me with no one with whom to share them.
Yet, Alzheimer's can also be a blessing.
As Al has drifted back in time,
I have seen glimpses of him that are new to me.

We had finished a round of errands
when I suggested going to Las Palomas for lunch.
Al's face lit up and he said,
"I wanted to suggest that but I thought it wasn't my place."

"My place!" What an epiphany!
I was being given a glimpse of Al as a child.
He must have controlled his world by always being in his place.
Al grew up in England during World War II,
with a mother who wanted to make everyone happy and a
brilliant alcoholic father.
I can see this little boy with his dog Nicky,
withdrawing into his proper place.

Al's place must have begun to change when he joined
the Royal Air Force after WWII.
He was sent to Egypt where he won the respect of his men by
knowing the length of the Queen Mary.
His place must have further expanded as he graduated
from Exeter College, Oxford, and won a scholarship
to the University of Texas.
Receiving his Ph.D. must have burst the cocoon, leaving him in the
place in which I joined him over forty hears ago.

Now as we go for ice cream or French fries, I better
understand who Alfie is because I now know him as three people:
  the child who knew his place,
  the vibrant dynamic man that I married, and
  the child to which Alzheimer's has returned him.

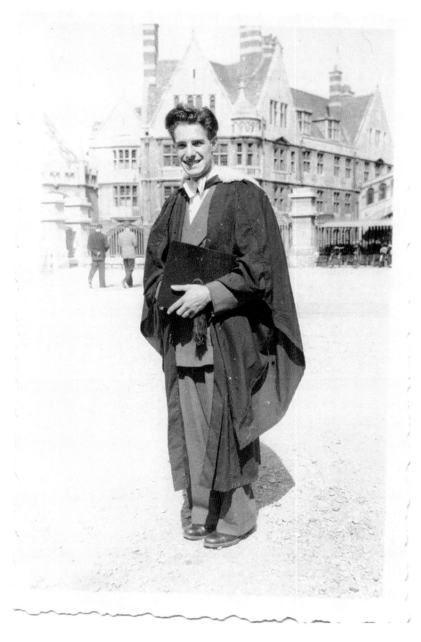

I Should Have Known

When Al left the department, after eight years of administration,
without staying to teach,
I should have known.

When Al started wanting to leave the symphony at intermission
and the opera before the last act,
I should have known.

When we went to Petit St. Vincent and he didn't snorkel
after arranging a snorkeling trip,
I should have known.

When Al became agitated when I went out in the evening,
I should have known.

When Al refused to do anything on the spur of the moment,
I should have known.

When Al refused to try a new restaurant,
I should have known.

When Al refused to drive at night even though his vision was
better than mine,
I should have known.

When Al stopped cooking,
I should have known.

When we went to Paris and spent most of the time in the apartment,
I should have known.

When Al bought books and never read them,
I should have known.

What should I have known?
That Al was frightened.

Frightened that he couldn't update his skills to teach even an
undergraduate class;
Frightened that he couldn't concentrate for so long at a time;
Frightened to do something new even though he wanted to do it;
Frightened to be alone;
Frightened of anything unplanned;

Frightened to try a new restaurant, where the place was unfamiliar;
Frightened of having to concentrate in night traffic;
Frightened of not remembering how to cook or even find a recipe in a cookbook;
Frightened of crowds of people in new places;
Frightened because he couldn't remember the previous paragraph (or sentence).

Why should such an intelligent, educated, sophisticated man be frightened?
Alzheimer's was robbing him of his memory, leaving him
in a world he didn't understand and thus couldn't control.
So he just avoided those situations that caused him distress.

He pulled the cocoon of his familiar controllable world, tighter and tighter around himself.
He didn't know why he acted as he did; he didn't know what had changed or that he had changed.
I should have known, but I didn't.

I do not feel guilty for not knowing.
I stopped trying to get him to "do something."
We left at intermission or before the last act.
I said I didn't really want to snorkel either.
The ladies started playing bridge at our house each week.
We politely declined spur of the moment invitations.
We always went to Jeffrey's, our favorite restaurant.
I drove at night.
I started to learn to cook.
We watched the French Open on television rather than see the sights of Paris.
I put the books quietly on the shelf.

Would I have behaved any differently if I had known that Alzheimer's was beginning its insidious journey, leaving him frightened and confused?
No, I think not.
Because I didn't know he was frightened, I didn't take away his dignity by reassuring him;
I didn't shatter his protective screen, which would only have left him exposed and vulnerable.

I should have known, but I'm glad I didn't.

Frisky

When people ask me "How is Al?"
I don't know how to answer.
Are they asking me about the vibrant,
articulate friend they remember?
If so, the question has no meaning;
he is no longer here.
Are they asking about the three-year old
I visit most days?
If so, the doctors are amazed at how well
he is doing.

If I ask him how he is,
he will reply with his new, favorite word: frisky.
He is feeling very frisky.
Then he will add "I am the most
fortunate person alive."

So rather than go into detail when
friends ask, I just say "Fine, thank you."

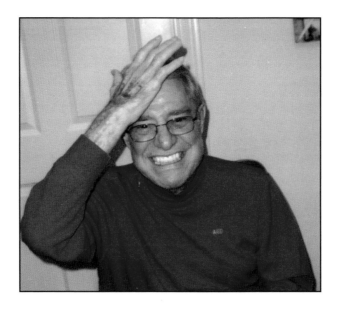

Lost in Time

Alfie, like any three-year old, loves to ride in the car.
He loves feeling the warm sun on his arms,
watching the puffy white clouds floating in the sky,
and especially seeing the crisscrossing contrails.

We go out for a drive almost every day.
Sometimes we go for ice cream,
sometimes for French fries,
sometimes to do errands,
sometimes just to ride around.

Our conversation varies little:
"You look beautiful."
"Thank you, Alfie."
"Where are we going?"
"For a ride."
"You look beautiful today."
"Thank you, love."
"Where are we going?"
"Would you prefer ice cream or French fries?"
"French fries. Did you know we've been married 44 years?"
"Yes, Alfie, we have been very lucky."
"You look beautiful today."

Then like a rainbow appearing after a raging storm,
Alfie suddenly smiles,
straightens his shoulders,
and looks and sounds like my wonderful
English-gentleman husband.
He is witty, charming, and articulate for a few minutes,
then like the rainbow, he fades away.
But it reminds me that he is there in my memory.
He is not gone; he is just lost in time.
I can always close my eyes and travel back to visit with him.

Yes, Alfie, 44 years is a long time; we have been blessed.

In God's Time

Al, my husband of 44 years, has Alzheimer's.
Don't turn away in fear or embarrassment.
He is not refusing to take a shower,
putting keys in the refrigerator,
wandering around barefoot in the rain, or
exhibiting any other odd behavior
often associated with Alzheimer's.
He just has no memory of people or events.

He loves having friends visit.
He doesn't remember them,
but he feels the warmth of their friendship.
He smiles and thanks them for coming
and suggests that they leave after about five minutes.

He loves to run errands with me.
We go by the laundry and the kids come to the car to say hello.
We go by the florist and the owner comes to the car with a gift.
We drive down MoPac Freeway and he comments that the
surface is so smooth.
We drive down Loop 360 and he points out the lovely views.
He never fails to marvel at the color of the blue sky
or smile every time he sees birds on a wire.

He remembers me, at least for the present.
He remembers that we have been married for 44 years.
Yet, I sometimes think I am not Nell the person to him,
but the sum of all those whom he has loved.
He sees me, and he is filled with love
and happiness and contentment and peace.

He is truly living in God's time:
He doesn't remember the past,
so he doesn't fret over past failures.

The future is an abstract concept, so he doesn't worry about it. He lives only in the present moment, a moving target of about thirty seconds.

Yes, Al is living in God's time.

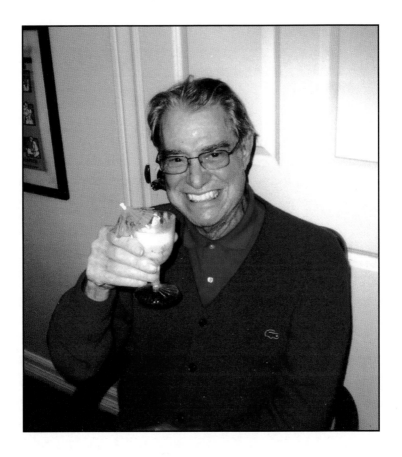

Where is Al?

"Where is Al tonight?"
asked an acquaintance at a concert.
Where is Al? I wish I knew.

He is physically tucked into bed at Barton House,
asleep like any three-year old should be.
But where is he mentally?
Is he really that happy child I visit so often?
Does he really love the sun and French fries and
riding in the car?

He has no memory of people and events,
so what does he think about?
Is his mind filled with blue sky and puffy clouds?
Does he smile in his sleep as he dreams about French fries?
Or is his mind empty, filled only with a web of
endless cotton candy?

Where is Al tonight? I don't know.
I only pray that he is content and not in anguish
over being trapped in the void of an empty mind.

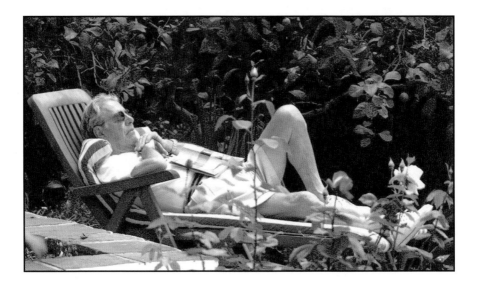

Tennis Balls

There is a graveyard for dead tennis balls behind court 13.
Some have participated in exciting matches;
some have been used by kids fooling around.
The balls rest silently in their gully,
unresponsive to the sun, wind, and rain
as their colors fade to grey.

An Alzheimer's home is a graveyard for people
for whom the past is dead.
Some have lived full, exciting lives; others have foolishly
played their lives away.
The residents sit patiently unresponsive to the world around
them as Alzheimer's takes their lives away

Do the tennis balls remember all the games won and lost?
Do the Alzheimer's patients mourn their memories lost?

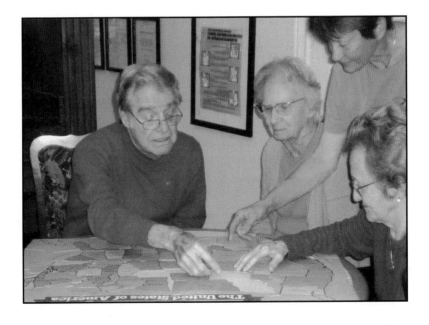

Why Should I?

I will not feel sorry for myself: Why should I?
I have been blessed with five loving, interesting children,
eight wonderful grandchildren, and many dear friends.
I have been blessed for over forty years with a husband I love
dearly.
I am now blessed with a charming three-year old
who needs my love and attention.

I will not feel sorry for myself: Why should I?
I love sitting on the terrace in the summer with a martini,
reading to the music of the fishpond waterfall.
I love sitting in the living room in the winter with a glass of wine,
reading to the music of the fire.
I love eating at the table with colorful linen, fresh flowers, and
sparkling silver.
I love saying the blessing and eating one of my experiments.

I will not feel alone: Why should I?
If I am alone, it will be by choice.
I will not sit at home waiting for someone to call.
If I want company, I will call a family member or a friend.
I may feel lonely, but I do not have to be alone.

I will not worry: Why should I?
I have enough money to keep Al in Barton House,
the place where he is sheltered, loved, and occupied.
I have enough money to continue with the charities that are
important to us.
I have enough money to buy three pairs of shoes and two shirts
any time I want.

I will not be bored: Why should I?
God gave me an inquiring mind,
a love of reading and music,
a passable backhand, and
the gift of new editions of my books always around the
corner.

Yet, self-pity is insidious.
It creeps in uninvited and often unrecognized.
Like the acute moments of grief by which I am
suddenly gripped,
self-pity unexpectedly grabs my heart and I am afraid.
Then my head takes control and I know in my heart
how truly blessed I have been.
I will not feel sorry for myself: Why should I?

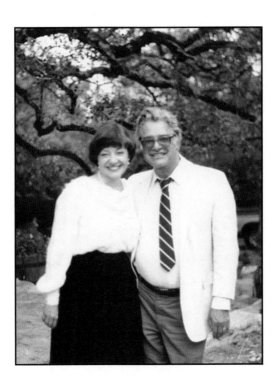

Gone

This All Saints Day I will remember my husband Al.
When did he die?
I don't remember exactly when it began but
it must have been a long time ago.
All I know now is that he is gone.

His brilliant mind – gone;
His penetrating ability to see through details – gone;
His strong leadership skills – gone;
His phenomenal vocabulary – gone;
His wonderful culinary creations – gone;
His unerring eye for style and beauty – gone;
His fluent German, French, Italian – gone;
His impeccable taste in art, music, and wine – gone;
His ability to charm all men and beasts – gone;

All gone to the ravages of Alzheimer's.

What remains?
A loving child with a beautiful smile,
who loves the sun, ice cream, French fries, and car rides.
His love of family also remains,
even if he doesn't always remember our names.

So next All Saints Day,
I will probably remember the passing of the child,
as Alzheimer's continues its relentless march.
Then on some future All Saints Day,
as the cycle of life closes,
I will remember the soul of my husband Al.

All Saints Day, 2007

I Don't Want to Go!

Al has been in an Alzheimer's home for eight months.
He is content, well taken care of by a loving staff.

For the first few months, I went every day.
I took him out for rides, ice cream, and French fries.
Then, I started taking a day off each week,
just to be me, not Al's wife.

After six months, I even gave myself a couple of days off.
I was learning more and more about who I was.
But we still went for rides, ice cream, and French fries.

It is getting harder and harder to visit him.
We are on our ninth month.

I have finally admitted to myself that there are times I don't
want to go.

I don't want to go!
I don't want to go!
I don't want to go!

BUT, he still recognizes me; his face lights up when he sees me.
Seeing me means rides, ice cream, and French fries.

So I will go.

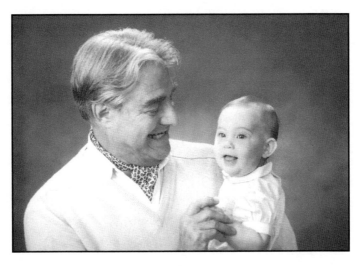

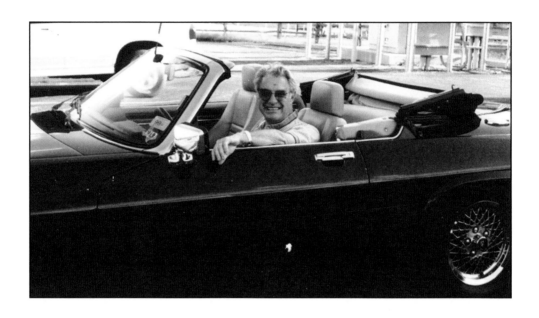

I Will Ask

I will not feel left out during holidays:
Why should I?
If I am not asked,
it will be because of miscommunication, not intent.
If I am not asked,
each child thinks another has.
If I am not asked, I will ask.
And I did.

Thanksgiving, 2007

Sudden Moments of Acute Grief

Just when I think I have everything under control,
some little something will happen and I am overwhelmed
with acute grief.

A Jag pulls up beside me with the sleek lines that Al loves.
I see his tennis racquet in my trunk and know he will never
play again.
It is "tini time" and Al isn't here to share a martini with me.
Al can sing all the words to "A Nightingale Sang in
Berkeley Square" but can't remember any details of our life
together.

The children are over for dinner and Al isn't sitting on the
middle step directing everyone.
My always immaculately dressed husband pees in his pants
and smiles and says, "It's ok."
I bring him something of his own and he says, "How thoughtful
of you."
Al smiles and says, "I adore you; do you know that?"
A notice comes from Barton House about the holiday festivities:
Bring a gift to open on Christmas morning—without me.
I decorate the tree alone: He didn't like to hang
ornaments, but he was always there before.

Thanksgiving and Al's birthday will be a piece of cake.
Christmas will be more difficult, like when I read the
lesson at the Midnight Service that Al has read for over fourty
years.

Can I do it without going to pieces? I don't know, but I'll try.

And a Little Child Shall Lead Them

After a hectic year, Christmas is approaching.
Colorful wrap litters the table and carols are playing.
Are we enjoying the music?
Probably not, we are too busy to hear.

While the traffic is snarled and our tempers are short,
Pop is content to ride in the car and enjoy the passing scene.

While unchosen and unbought gifts cloud our minds with worry,
Pop marvels at a flawless, clear blue sky.

While we scurry around too tired even to enjoy the season,
Pop sees birds on a wire and says, "That makes my day."

While we worry about Christmas dinner and all the fixings,
Pop looks forward to a snack of French fries.

While we greet friends and acquaintances alike with a
meaningless kiss,
Pop says, "I adore you; do you know that?"

May we learn from Pop to treasure the really important things
in life:
love, family, health, and the little blessings we receive every day.

Christmas, 2007

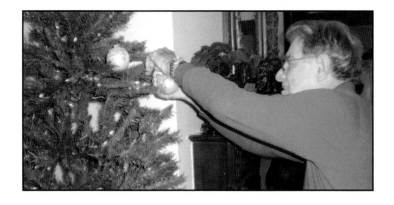

January

In January of 1990, Al had major surgery to remove a polyp from his colon.

In January of 2005, Al had major surgery to remove a polyp from his colon.

In January of 2007, Al had major surgery to remove a kidney.

I am not superstitious but I dread January of 2008.
I have come to terms with Al's Alzheimer's,
but I panic at the thought of his having to go back into the hospital.

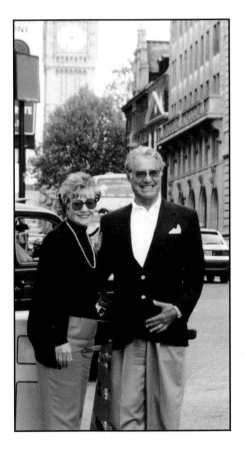

Moments in the Sun

When we met, Al was a confident young man,
just leaving the cocoon of graduate school and
moving into the academic world as a professor.
He grew in stature and confidence,
becoming a leader in the field of computer science.
In all that he did, he maintained that gloss of the English gentleman.

Oh, sure, he was cross and grumpy at times,
usually around 5 o'clock.
One of the kids would run get him a snack,
to raise his blood sugar, and normalcy would return.

As the Alzheimer's began its insidious takeover,
Al became more passive, yet agitated with
any deviation to his routine.
His world began to shrink, as the family learned to
accommodate his changing moods.

Then the day came when we could no longer
deny that Al had a problem.
And our days were highlighted with French fries
and moments in the sun.

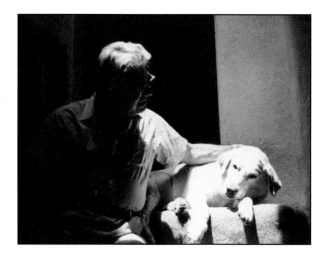

Shirts

The last time I counted, Al had over 70 shirts:
White shirts,
Blue shirts,
Striped shirts,
Checkered shirts,
Long-sleeved shirts,
Short-sleeved shirts,
Silk shirts,
Cotton shirts.

They have now gone to Goodwill in two batches.
The first was soon after he moved into Barton House,
when I divided them into wearable and not wearable.
The second has gone today.

Why now? It is the beginning of winter.
Al is always cold;
he huddles in a sweater over a long sleeved knit shirt.
I now understand that he will never again wear a crisp,
starched, white shirt, a lovely silk guayabera,
or his lemon shirt from St. Kitts.

My hope is that someone else this holiday season
will dress up to the nines in one of Al's beautiful shirts
to celebrate the holiday season.
A shirt is meant to be worn,
not hang in solitary splendor in a closet.

Only, I didn't give away the lemon shirt;
I will have it remade to fit me.

Tini Time

Alcohol has always been part of the fabric of our family life.
In the early days, a bottle of rum (for daiquiris) and a bottle of
bourbon (for Manhattans) were staples in our weekly shopping
cart.

Then we moved to gin and 6 o'clock became known as "tini" time.
Tini time meant more than drinking martinis:
It represented the time when the family gathered
together in the kitchen to cook, talk, and catch up on the day's
happenings.

Tini time was family time.

As we grew older, Al became an adventurous cook and
connoisseur of wine.
Julia, Marcella, Pierre, Craig, and Jacques became his favorite
authors.

Tini time became a serious business.

I was relegated to peeling vegetables and making the salad.
We began a Gourmet Group with friends,
and experimented with ever-more-challenging recipes
and unfamiliar wines.
I only did the prep work and just knew that I liked red wine
better than white.

Al and I loved to travel.
Each trip was highlighted by the food and wine.
We ate pub food and drank lager in London;
we people-watched and drank champagne at
sidewalk cafes in Paris.
We drank martinis in Harry's Bar and red wine in the Piazza San
Marco.

I have now lost my tini-time partner and traveling companion;

I must rethink the role of food and drink in my life.
I can't live on salads and Lean Cuisines.
I can't use martinis to dull the ache of loss.
Of course, I can always visit one of the children for their
tini times.
All five of them have carried on the tradition;
all five are super cooks and know their wines.

I can also visit dear friends for their tini times.

But ultimately, I must learn to handle tini time by myself.
So I am learning to cook and limiting my martinis.
I am taking small steps like
buying a bottle of Kendall Jackson chardonnay.
And eventually maybe the Gourmet Group will assign me
something other than salads.

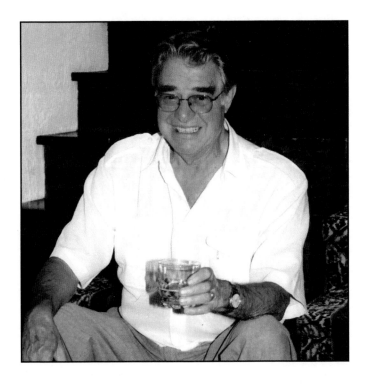

Articles

Friends and family keep sending me articles about Alzheimer's,
hoping to encourage me.

There are three kinds of articles:
The first describes an alternative-medicine miracle cure reported
by a "doctor" using one or two "cures" as proof.
To me as a scientist, these articles are good for a laugh,
but I am appalled that people actually believe them.

The second reports on a breakthrough in cell or gene research that
bodes well for a future cure, but probably not in our lifetime.

The third reports on this or that current new drug that
purports to help restore memory.
It is this third type that looks helpful, but is it really?

What does it mean to "restore memory"?
Does it mean that short-term memory improves?
Does it mean that forgotten people and places from the past are
now remembered?
To what point on the continuum of memory does it restore someone?

My husband is living the contented life of a three-year old.
He is in a wonderful assisted-living facility for Alzheimer's
patients, where he is cared for by a loving staff
who understand the disease.
I take him out for car rides, French fries, and afternoon tea.
What would it mean to him if his memory improved?

He now describes himself as frisky, ready to live another ten years:
If his memory improved,
would he remember that he has only one kidney,
heart trouble, type II diabetes, and lung disease?

He loves his small room, painted a light blue,
with his favorite pictures on the wall
and his stuffed Labrador on the bed:
If his memory improved,
would he remember his lovely Westlake home and feel cheated?

He was a gourmet chef:
If his memory improved,
would he disdain the simple meals he now enjoys?

He loves to go to the Steeping Room for tea and cucumber
sandwiches:
If his memory improved,
would his pleasure fade in the memories of tea at the Savoy?

He was always impeccably dressed:
If his memory improved,
would his bouts of incontinence humiliate him?

If his memory improved,
he might remember the names of his children,
grandchildren,
and friends;
he might remember that he was once a great scientist.

Remembering might make his family and friends happy.
But would it benefit Al?
I think not; even Alzheimer's patients have to live in the now.
He is better off content in the present, with few memories,
than he would be living in the present, remembering the past.

Friends and family,
please don't send me any more articles on Alzheimer's.

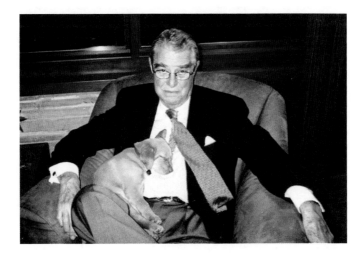

Grieve

My goldfish has vanished, the big one that has survived so much.
I know what this means:
He is gone forever and I grieve.
Silly to grieve for a fish, but I do.

My husband has Alzheimer's.
I know what this means:
He is here, but gone forever,
And I grieve.
Silly to grieve for someone who is still here, but I do.

Is it really silly? Maybe not.
My drinking buddy, companion, and best friend is gone.
What's left in his place is a small child in the body of a grown man.
So I grieve.
His body is here, but he's gone:
The essence of who he was is gone.
So I grieve.

When a loved one dies, we grieve for the person.
When a loved one has Alzheimer's, we grieve for the past.
So I mourn for both my husband and my fish.

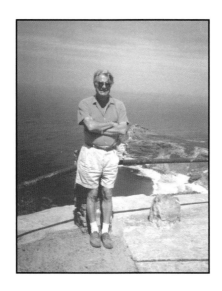

Ink

After Al had been in an Alzheimer's home for a year,
I adopted a couple of four-week-old, black fluff balls.
They were identical black-smoke tabby kittens.
Except, one had a little white spot on his chest.
I called them Ink and Spot.
I killed Ink.

I loved to see them romp around the room,
jumping from table top to table top.
They were tireless—and indistinguishable,
unless you picked one up and looked at his chest.
I killed Ink.

They grew and grew and grew, looking more alike each day.
They purred in concert and graduated to dry food.
When they were fourteen-and-a-half weeks old,
I killed Ink.

I didn't mean to.
I was folding laundry and tossed a sheet back into the dryer
because it wasn't dry.
I didn't see Ink slip into the dryer while I was folding sheets.
I turned on the dryer.
I killed Ink.

Oh, God, I heard a thump and thought the dryer was off balance.
Why oh why didn't I go back and check?
I'd pulled him out of the open dryer before.
Why oh why didn't I go back and check?
I killed Ink.

When I found him, I clutched him to my chest
and screamed and screamed and screamed.
He didn't revive and neither have I.
I killed Ink.

It was an accident, but I killed Ink.
I know it was an accident, but I killed him.

Change in Pronouns

Our outings have changed slightly over the last few months.
Al is "off" ice cream, so French fries it is.
Our conversations still vary little, but the focus has changed.

"I adore you; do you know that?"
"Yes, Alfie, I know."
"I adore you, Nellie; do you know that?"
"Yes, Alfie, you just told me."
"Oh, I'm sorry."
"What would I do without you?"
"You'll never have to find out."
"I adore you; do you know that?"

I wonder what Al's change from "you" in "You are beautiful"
to "I" in "I adore you" means?
Is he getting more in touch with his feelings? Probably not.
Introspection is an exercise in abstract thinking,
one of the skills that Alzheimer's steals from its victims.
Is his world constricting,
so that only his inner feelings remain?
Oh, he still says I look beautiful when I arrive, but he does not
repeat the phrase as a mantra anymore.
It is almost as if what is beautiful now is the outing that I represent.

Probably the change in pronouns means nothing.
That is one of the problems with having a loved one with Alzheimer's:
We try too hard to interpret the uninterpretable.
It is all we have left.

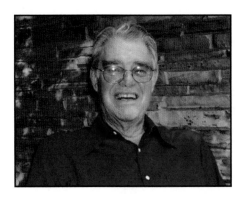

We Are Alone

My mother used to talk about two types of widows:
grass and sod.
The grass widow is divorced;
the sod widow's husband is dead.
Both are alone.

There should be a third kind of widow:
The Alzheimer's widow.
Our husbands are no longer with us; the bodies survive but the
souls and essence of our husbands have been
replaced by the innocence of a child.
We are alone.

We are in limbo; we are technically married
but are, in fact, single.
The men that we married are no longer with us.
The men that we lived with, worked with, played with,
had children with, are gone.
In their places are children who need the same time and attention
as our other children did.
Only this time, our husbands are not there to give help and support
because they are the children.
We are alone.

The marriage relationship of an Alzheimer's widow and her husband
is as irrevocably severed as a marriage ended by death or divorce.
We are alone.
We grieve for our marriages and our departed husbands.
We love the child, but our husband and marriage are gone.
We are alone.

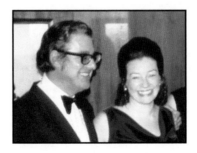

Blessed

At tennis this morning, we decided that nurture beats nature:
As we get another year older, our tennis games just get better.
We all expressed our gratitude for good things that life has given us.
A few minutes later my partner came over and said she realized
that not all of us were equally lucky.
It took me a minute to realize that she was referring to Al's
Alzheimer's.

Oh no, I thought: Of all people I am the most fortunate.
I had forty wonderful years with the man I loved.
True, in the last five years, I have watched my husband regress
into the child of my old age.
But he is now contentedly living in a warm, safe environment.
I can take him out for French fries or tea, watch him marvel at
the blue sky, the clouds, and the birds on a wire.
I can hear him happily sing along with the CD, remembering all
the words.
I am so fortunate to be able to afford such loving care for my
child/husband.

I am fortunate to have a blended family with five wonderful children.
They are all so different, yet so loving and supportive.
I have been blessed with five very distinctive in-laws.
We all have such a good time together, eating, drinking, and
laughing.

I am fortunate to have eight grandchildren and one great-grandchild.
They are as different and interesting as their parents.
It has been a delight to watch them grow into distinctly different
individuals.
Who knows, they may change the world.

I have tennis friends, bridge friends, church friends, old friends,
new friends.
I have books to write; I have songs to sing.
I have a house I love with a kitty to greet me when I come home.

Less fortunate than others?
Absolutely not!

Renee

Renee died last night.
Another Barton House angel has been set free.

I didn't know Renee before Alzheimer's robbed her of her mind,
but I know a lot about her.
Her clear sweet gaze reflected her early beauty.
The sparkle in her blue eyes spoke of a lively personality.
The devotion of her daughter tells of her success as a mother.

I shall miss Renee.
I have seen her four or five times a week for 16 months.
I remember when she patted Al's hand during the last
Halloween party.
I remember her daughter going through magazines with her.
I remember her trying to get into Al's room and his saying, "Boom."

I wish I had known her before the ravages of Alzheimer's sent
her to Barton House,
but I am glad that I had the privilege of knowing her there.

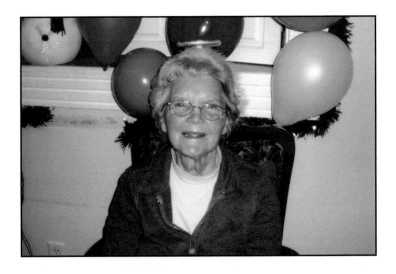

Blindsided by a Melody

I was blindsided by a melody last night.

The orchestra was playing old love songs
and I cried.
Couples were holding hands in front of me
and I cried.
I don't want people to feel sorry for me
but I cried.

Our forty-fifth wedding anniversary is tomorrow
and I will cry.
All that remains of those forty-five years
are memories and an 80-year-old child who likes French fries.

My husband has Alzheimer's and
I live in two parallel universes:
the everyday present with my memories
and a man/child who loves French fries.

I don't grieve for the past or the child,
but I do fear that memories of the child
will overshadow the memories of the man.

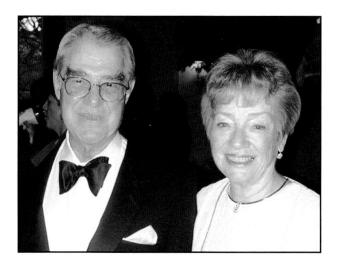

Blindsided by a Picture

An old graduate student of my husband's called when she
heard he was ill.
She remembered him fondly and wanted to be sure he
was in a good place.
She promised to send photos of him signing her master's
thesis.

The pictures arrived on my computer yesterday;
I was in tears.

Living in the world of Alzheimer's,
I had forgotten how handsome Al was.
I had forgotten what lovely silver hair he had.
I had forgotten how well he always dressed.
I had forgotten how he loved his bright ties.
I had forgotten how his presence dominated his office.
I had forgotten the essence of this wonderful man.

As I live with the child that Alzheimer's has given me,
I must remember to remember the man who he was.

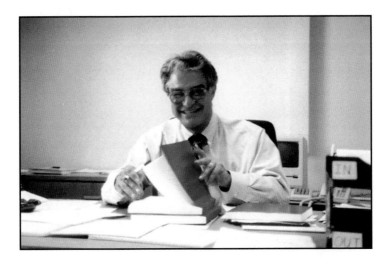

Loneliest Night of My Life

Election night 2008 was the loneliest night of my life.
My husband Al has been in an Alzheimer's home for a year
and a half.
I have been prepared for holidays, birthdays, and other
special occasions.
I made sure that I was surrounded by family and friends.

As the election approached, I thought about voting for Al.
I had his voter registration, and I knew how he would want to vote.
Yet, I couldn't do that.
So I voted early and waited with anticipation for election night.

I was prepared to spend the evening relishing the results as they
came in and enjoying a good bottle of wine.
But I wasn't prepared for the overwhelming sense of grief and
loss I felt when he wasn't here to share the Obama
victory with me.

For over forty years, we have shared such moments together.
Oh, I do miss him so.

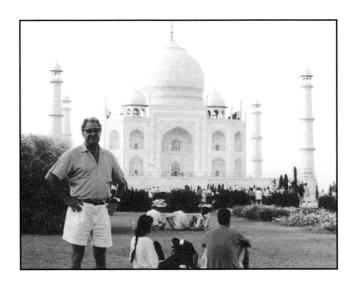

Forgotten Facts

Al remembers almost nothing about the present or the past.
Alzheimer's has robbed him of those memories along with
his ability to think abstractly.

So I was delighted when on one of our outings he kept
repeating Obama, Obama, Obama.
Wonderful, I thought.
His love of politics was still smoldering somewhere in his brain.

The day after the election, we went for a drive.
I told him excitedly that Obama had won.
"Won what?" he asked.
"The Presidency," I replied.
"Of what?" he asked.
"Of the United States," I replied.
"What's his experience?" he asked.
"He was a senator from Illinois," I replied.
"Senator—whatever that is," he said.

Obama wasn't a name to him; it was a nonsense phrase
he had seen on yard signs.
His repeating it had meant nothing.
I should have known better, but
I so wanted him to share the joy of this election with me.

But I have learned something: Alzheimer's marches on.
He is forgetting the meanings of words now.
"Senator—whatever that is."

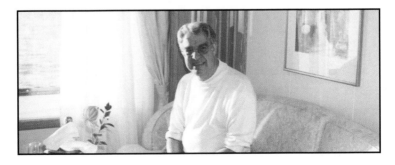

Stuffed Animals

Most Alzheimer's patients relate to stuffed animals.
Miss Nancy, in particular, loved stuffed animals.
She always walked around Barton House,
carrying one, and often two, with her.

In fact, she daily went into other residents' rooms
and borrowed theirs.
At the end of the day, one of the loving staff
would tuck her in, tell her good night, and
return the animals to their rightful owners.
Occasionally, Miss Nancy would exchange
animals, borrowing one and substituting another.

My husband loved his two stuffed Labrador dogs,
one brown and one yellow.
Miss Nancy would borrow them on a regular basis
and they would be returned each evening,
sometimes accompanied by a dog of a different origin.

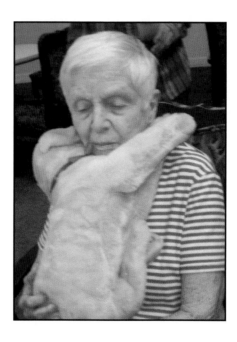

When my husband died, we donated his stuffed dogs to Miss Nancy's
permanent collection.

Parallel Universe

Thank you, Tony, for your words of comfort, support, and assurance.
You wanted me to know that there is a world for me when my
husband concedes the battle to Alzheimer's.
I know, Tony, because I am half in that world;
I live in parallel universes.

One is Barton House, the Alzheimer's facility that has become
home to Al.
This universe is made up of car rides, French fries, and tea with
cucumber sandwiches.
This is the universe in which I reside with my husband/child.

The other is the expanding world in which I am learning to function.
It is made up of work, choir, tennis, bridge, learning to cook,
dinner with friends.
This is the universe in which I reside alone.

At first, the Alzheimer's world was the only one I knew.
Then slowly, I tried to navigate the waters of the new world.
As time has gone by, I have moved more and more into this
strange, new world.

Now I inhabit both worlds.
I live a schizophrenic life straddling the line between them.
I only hope that I have as much grace making this transition
as Al has shown making the transition into his new world.

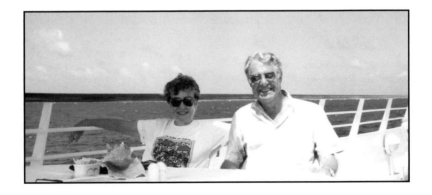

Panic

Al has been in a wonderful Alzheimer's facility for a year and a half.
I have lived in fear that something would happen, that he
couldn't stay.

Every time I got a call from Barton House, I was afraid
something had happened,
that I would have to move him.
From the first, I knew Barton House was the safe, warm,
loving place that he needed.
He was at home.

And they did call about some behavior or another,
touching inappropriately,
getting angry at someone who wanted to come into his room,
asking the ladies if he could kiss them,
not wanting to take a shower.
Each time I panicked.
Each time the problem was solved.

The new hospice nurse warned me that as Alzheimer's relentless
march continues, Al might need to be moved to a skilled
nursing facility.
This time I didn't panic.
When/if that time comes, he will no longer need his
Barton House home.
I no longer need to react like a mother tiger protecting her young.
Barton House has served its purpose.
When/if that time comes, he will be near the end of this
terrible journey and finally going home.

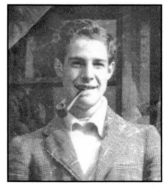

Am I Competent?

On a recent drive, after struggling for words, Al said,
"Am I competent?"
I responded, "Of course you are."
He repeated the question and I repeated my answer.

He repeated it a third time,
and I assured him that he had always been a most competent person.
After the fourth time, I asked him what he meant by competent.
He said, "Can I cope?"

I reassured him again and asked if he was worried about
something.
He said no, he was very peaceful.

Was I answering the wrong question?
In his Alzheimer's-altered mind, just what was he really asking me?
Was he asking me if he were competent to take the next step?
Was he asking me if he could cope with dying?

I turn the question inward: How well will I cope with his dying?

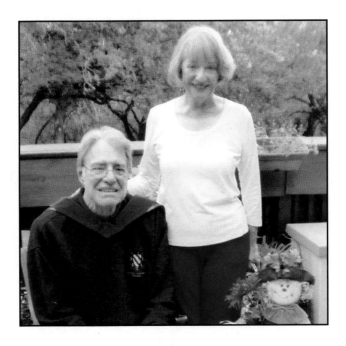

Al Took Charge

On the Thursday before Al died,
he told two of his children that
he was "negotiating to be misplaced;"
he was going home.

On Friday morning,
he removed all the pictures from his wall and
placed his books on the table,
ready to take home.

He went to the nursing station and
asked for his bill.
The administrator wrote him one for $100,
which he signed.

He went to his room and went to bed.
He was going home.

He roused on Sunday to say "Amen!"
in a loud voice as he received communion.
He closed his eyes and went to a place we could not follow.
He was going home.

He died peacefully on that next Tuesday evening,
surrounded by his family.
We drank a champagne toast to our husband and father.
He was home.

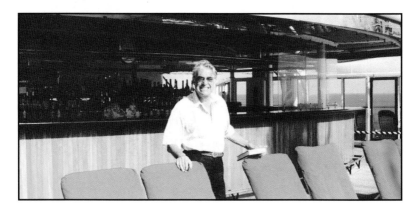

Freedom

Al is free.
Free of the Alzheimer's that robbed him of his mind.
Free of the aging body that let him down in the end.
Free to soar with his beloved birds in a clear blue sky.

Al is free.

We are free.
Free to say goodbye to the wounded child he had become.
Free to remember the wonderful English gentleman he was.
Free to welcome back the memory of our husband and father.

We are free.

Thanks be to God.

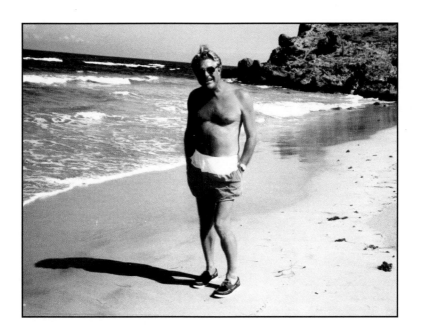

Is It Inappropriate?

My husband has died of Alzheimer's after a long struggle,
and I am relieved.

He is no longer the helpless child I took for French fries,
and I am happy.

He is no longer bound to the body that was failing him,
and I am joyful.

People come up and say that they know I am grieving.
I grieved when he was in the hospital so long.
I grieved a little each day that I visited him over the last
two years.
I grieved each time I saw something that reminded me of the real Al.
I am not grieving now, for he is free.
I am relieved, happy, joyful, and content.
I no longer have to worry about him;
I can just enjoy the memories of happier times.

Al is free, and so am I.

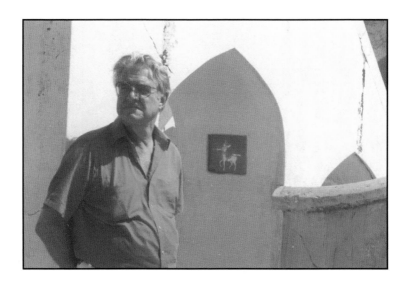

My Mind Is Wandering

They were such lovely flowers.
I wonder who sent them?
Oh, where am I?
I remember;
I'm playing tennis.

It was wonderful to see
old friends at the memorial service.
Oh dear, I missed the ball;
I must concentrate.
I'm playing tennis.

My mind is flitting back and forth
over the last ten days: Images
keep running through my mind.
Oh, I missed another volley;
I must remember to concentrate.
I'm playing tennis.

Who brought that wonderful cake?
I must remember to find out and thank them.
Oh, I double-faulted: what's the score?
Why is my mind wandering?
I should concentrate on tennis.

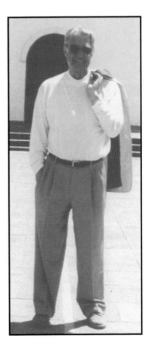

Everyone has been so kind and
said such nice things about my husband.
Earlier memories of happier times
are flooding back into my mind.
Oh, I missed another forehand;
We lost the match.
We've finished playing tennis.

Why is my mind wandering so?

Looking Up

Four months after my husband died of Alzheimer's,
I was feeling tired, with no energy.
I had a chapter to edit and shelves to clean;
still I just sat.

I went into my office and sat at the computer.
I felt so small and insignificant,
incapable of doing anything as I looked up at the screen.

Up at the screen?
My office chair was set at the lowest setting;
I *was* looking up at the screen.
I raised my chair and went to work.

That chair will always be a metaphor to me
of raising up and just doing something.
Making a beginning.

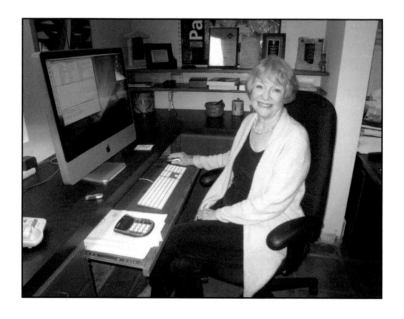

Why Can't I Cry?

When my husband was diagnosed with Alzheimer's,
I cried.

When he was in the hospital for so long,
I cried.

When he went into Barton House,
I cried.

When I would visit him in Barton House,
I often cried on the way home.

Now that he is free,
I haven't cried.

When my cat was gone for two days,
I cried.

My husband has been gone for six weeks.
Yet, I haven't cried.

Why can't I cry?
I won't be truly free until I can cry.

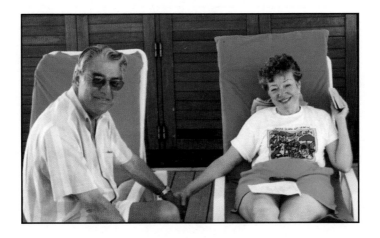

I Finally Cried

For six months after my husband's death from Alzheimer's,
I couldn't cry.

I finally broke down and cried on All Saints Day,
after a small, quiet, candle-light service at church.
I came home, lit a fire, had a glass of wine, and cried.

After a while, I went upstairs to get a photograph
album with which to reminisce.
I didn't choose photos from one of our many travels;
I chose the album of pictures taken at Barton House.

I realized then that it was the child for whom I was crying,
not my husband.
I was saying goodbye to the child who loved French fries,
cucumber sandwiches, and birds on a wire.

As I cried, the figure of the child was fading away;
the figure of my husband was emerging from the shadows.
I am now free to remember him as he really was,
the wonderful, kind, English gentleman I married.

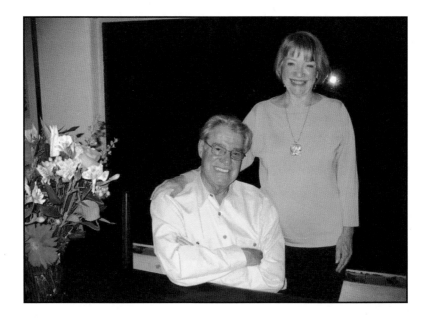

Grackles & Dragonflies

The Al of our early years didn't care much for birds.
By the middle years, he hung a bird feeder but usually
forgot to fill it.
By the time Alzheimer's had returned him to childhood,
he loved birds.
Seeing birds on a wire made our daily drive a success.
He particularly loved grackles.

After his death, I started saying hello to each grackle I saw.
Each one became a symbol of the Al-child of the later years.
I needed something concrete to bring back the old Al.
He loved cooking, but I couldn't say hello to a steak.

Then on the tennis court one morning, I saw a small flight
of dragonflies:
Beautiful, graceful, elegant dragonflies.
I knew I had my symbol.
I can't escape the scruffy, erasable grackles that are
everywhere,
but I search my garden every morning and evening,
looking for that beautiful, elusive dragonfly: my dearest Al.

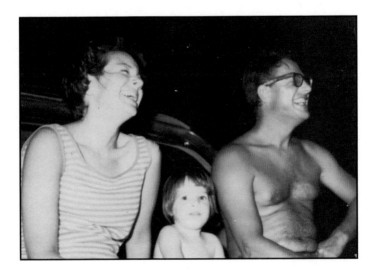

Thank You, Spot

When I came home from church, there was a message
telling me that my black kitty had been hit and killed by a car.
I went to pieces and sobbed and sobbed.

I didn't go to pieces when my husband was diagnosed with
Alzheimer's.
I didn't go to pieces when my husband had to go into an
Alzheimer's facility.
I didn't go to pieces when my husband died.
Why did the death of my kitty affect me so?

I was prepared for my husband's diagnosis;
I knew something was wrong.
I was prepared for the time when I couldn't take care of him
at home.
I was prepared for his death.
I was not prepared for the sudden death of my kitty.

When I had time to prepare,
I could be strong and control my emotions.
I didn't have time to prepare for kitty's death,
so I lost control.
Loss of control can sometimes be a blessing.
My sobs were not just for the loss of my kitty,
but for all the losses of the last few years.
I had cried for the loss of my child,
but I had not cried for the loss of my husband.
I feel better now that I have allowed myself to completely lose
control and truly grieve for the passing of Al and our life together.
Thank you my beloved kitty, for your life and your death.
God bless you.

Spot is now buried in the Dale pet cemetery along with his brother
Ink. In the future, I will get a marker for the graves of my two little
black fluff balls.

Easter Island

There were two places that Al particularly wanted to see:
St. Helena and Easter Island.
We traveled to St. Helena but not to Easter Island.

Somewhere in his Alzheimer's distorted mind,
he remembered that he wanted to see Easter Island.
He kept asking over and over when we were going.

I asked him why he wanted to go.
He said there were things to see.
Finally, I said, sure let's go.
He asked when?
I said on my birthday.

Every week or so, he would bring it up.
He asked how we would get there.
I said by plane to Chile and by boat from there.
He would ask, "Have we booked?"
Yes, Alfie, we have booked.
"Good," he would say.

After my birthday passed,
we were going on his birthday.
When his birthday passed,
we were going on my birthday.
These discussions gave him great pleasure
and the trip was always new in his mind.

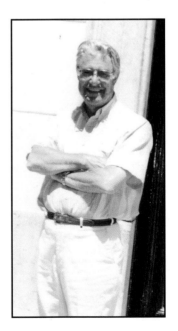

Al will never travel to Easter Island,
but I will take some of his ashes
and scatter them there.

Obituary for Alfred George Dale:
November 23, 1926 — May 5, 2009

"Our Father, we thank thee for these and all your blessings: our children, grandchildren, friends, creatures, and all the other blessings of this life."

The core of this blessing was said everyday in the Dale household for over 45 years, adding those for whom we were thankful as they came along. Al Dale lived his life counting his blessings.

He was born in Stoke-on-Trent, England, in 1926, the son of Alfred John and Marjorie Thomas Dale. He graduated from Wolstanton Grammar School and Exeter College, Oxford. Between high school and college he served in the British Air Force in Egypt, during the birth of Israel when everyone was shooting at the British. As a result, he never sat in a restaurant with his back to the door.

Following his graduation from Oxford in 1951, he came to the United States on a Smith-Mundt fellowship to study at The University of Texas. As he liked to say, "I liked Austin, so I stayed." He taught statistics in the Business School while a graduate student and received his Ph.D. in 1961. He was Chief of Applications and Theoretical Groups at the Linguistics Research Center for two years until the Computer Sciences Department was formed at UT, at which time he became one of the founding members of this new department.

During his long and illustrious career at UT, he also taught in the School of Library Science, served as a Research Scientist at the Computation Center, and was Associate Director of the Institute for Computing Science and Computer Applications. He served as Chairman of the CS Department twice and was closely involved with bringing Microelectronics and Computer Technology Corporation (MCC) to Austin. He retired in 1992 as Regents Professor Emeritus. He then went on to found and direct the Software Quality Institute until 1996.

Al supervised nine dissertations in the new field of computing and served on countless other dissertation and master's committees. He and his wife, Nell, often worked together in the early years and among his numerous papers were six co-authored with Nell.

Al was one of the cofounders of MRI Systems Corporation, one of the first software companies in Austin. He was a technical advisor for the United Nations in Bratislava and spent almost three years as Director of the United Nations Development Program's International Computer Education Center in Budapest, Hungary. He reviewed UNDP computing research programs in Israel, the Philippines, and India. He was National Science Foundation representative to the Soviet Academy of Sciences in the Collaborative US-USSR program on Scientific and Technical Cooperation in the Field of Applications of Computers to Management.

The family once asked Al of what he was most proud. His list included speaking fluent German and French and passable Italian, Russian, Czech, and Hungarian; cooking gourmet meals, especially leg of lamb; being involved with the founding of MRI; being instrumental in bringing MCC to Austin; and attending his beloved Exeter College, Oxford.

Al was also much involved with his church (St. Michael's Episcopal Church), serving as Senior Warden twice and reading the Old Testament lesson on Christmas Eve for over 40 years. He loved classical music and never missed a symphony concert or opera performance. He had impeccable taste in clothing, food, and wine. He loved to shop for Nell and prepare gourmet meals for his family and friends. He loved to travel and sit in sidewalk cafes around the world absorbing the atmosphere.

But most of all, Al loved his family: his wife, colleague, and best friend Nell; his children Judith Dale and her husband Philip Vitek, June Dale Gormley and her husband John, Robert Dale and his wife Maricarmen, Susan Dale Toth and her husband Christopher, and Sarah Dale Anderson and her husband Jim; his grandchildren Jimmie, Kate, Alex, Becca, Lila, Christopher, John Robert, and Kit;

his great granddaughter Sage; Al's first wife Elizabeth Dale, who attended all the family gatherings in the later years; and the Labrador dogs from Nicky to Winston, who gave him such joy.

The family wishes to express their gratitude to Dr. Anthony Aventa, Al's favorite doctor, our Hospice Austin team, and the staff at Barton House, an Alzheimer's home where Al spent his last two years being lovingly cared for.

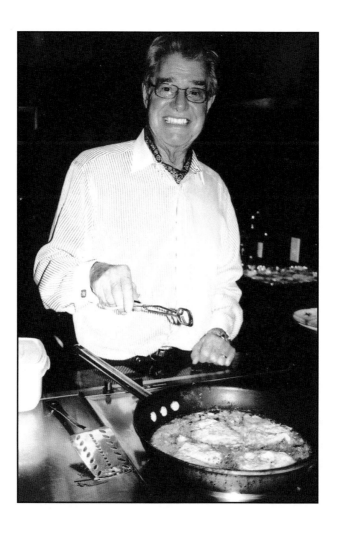

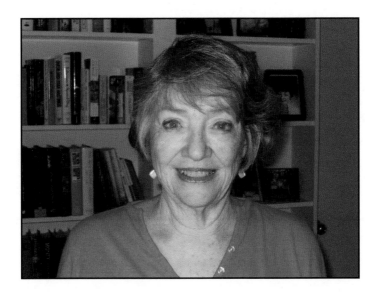

Dr. Nell B. Dale was one of the first women to get a Ph.D. in Computer Science in the early 1970s. She graduated from the University of Texas Department of Computer Sciences and remained on the faculty until her retirement from full-time teaching in 2000. She was originator and director of the Women in Science Program in the early '80s and has been a mentor to students and colleagues throughout her career. Her research interests have focused on computer science education as an academic discipline, having cochaired five dissertations in the area. During her career she has authored or coauthored 18 textbooks, many in multiple editions.

Dr. Dale has received the prestigious SIGCSE Award for Outstanding Contributions to Computer Science Education and was the first woman to receive the Association for Computing Machinery (ACM)'s prestigious Karl V. Karlstrom Outstanding Educator Award. She has won two Hamilton Awards for the best textbook published at UT in a given year. She has received the ABACUS Award from Upsilon Pi Epsilon, Honor Society for the Computing Sciences and was elected a Fellow of the ACM. She received a Doctor of Science, honoris causa, from Sewanee, The University of the South.

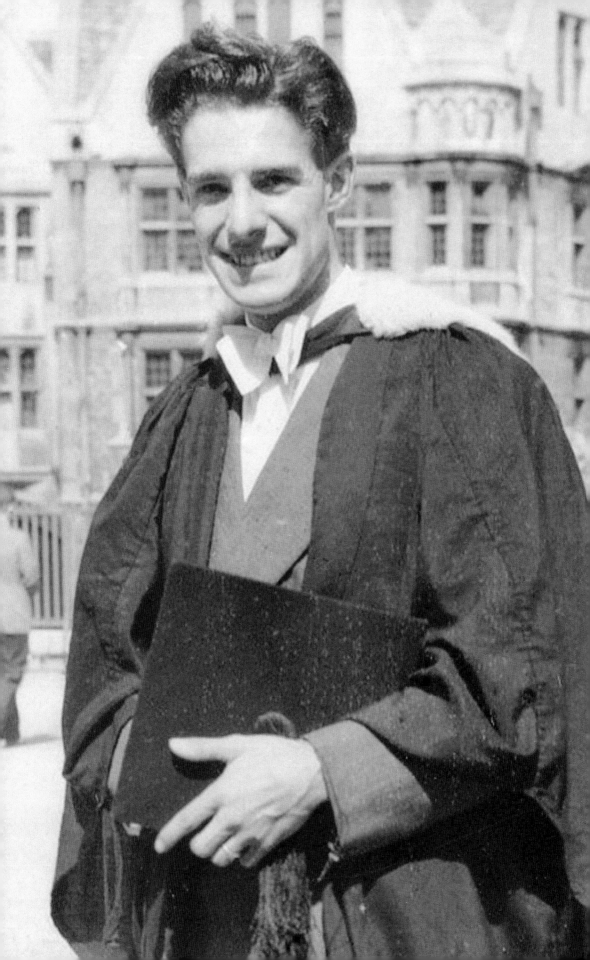

To my friends

So many of you wrote loving notes, remembering Al over the years. Your notes touched my heart and renewed forgotten memories.

After years of Alzheimer's I had forgotten the little things:
> *How he always supported me in whatever I wanted to do*
> *How he loved to buy clothes for me from the Neiman Marcus catalogue*
> *How he watched baseball with me even though he hated it*
> *How he dazzled everyone with his extraordinary vocabulary*
> *How he corrected our daughter's English teacher's spelling*
> *How he loved all creatures, big and small*
> *How he supported all those with whom he worked, from students to colleagues*
> *How he always had a kind word for everyone, but didn't suffer fools lightly*
> *How he loved me unconditionally*

Thank you all for reminding me of why I married this wonderful man.

Nell Dale